Dedications

This story would not be complete without mentioning all the important people that supported us along the way. Each and everyone of you made this possible.

To my husband Andrew, I know how hard it must have been for you to watch your mom die this way, but you stayed by her side the entire time. You truly are a loving and caring son, husband and friend.

To Mom's grandchildren, Misha, Kendra, Andrew, Laura, Chance and Raevyn, much gratitude for all the times you stopped in to stay so we could leave the house on occasion. You will never know how much it meant to us.

To Mom's beautiful sister, Irene, who visited as often as possible. Always making mom beam with delight to see you and chat with you about old times and family. Mom didn't remember much but she always remembered you :)

To all of Mom's nieces and nephews, godchildren and church children. You know who you are but too plentiful to list. It would certainly take a whole other book to recount all of the love, prayers and support that was shown along our journey. We are forever grateful.

To my best friend, Renie, who listened to countless daily stories of poop and other tattered tales, but always took my call, provided her home as a get away and stayed my friend even though I was often unavailable.

To my sisters, Linda and Georgia, for being there for me and understanding how much this had to do with caring for our own mother during her illness and how caring for my mother-in-law was filling my soul and changing me as a person. And, of course, for listening to yet more poop stories. I love you both so much.

To Mom's medical/hospice team, each and every one of you treated Mom with dignity and care.

And last but not least, I have to give a huge shout out to God, Joyce Meyer Ministries and Ellen DeGeneres.

To Joyce Meyer for reminding me daily that God loves me and this is what he wants me to do at this time. Also, that the mind is a battlefield and it's up to you what you choose to think about. "Where the mind goes, the man follows." (Proverbs 23:7)

To Ellen DeGeneres for making me laugh and sometimes cry everyday at 3:00pm. Being stuck at home most of the time, it was refreshing to see good people doing good things for others. I definitely look forward to your show everyday….thank you!

To God, I looked to you when I needed you most and true to your word…..you were there! Sometimes you think you may be lost then you realize you are exactly where you are suppose to be!

FROM CORPORATE TO CAREGIVER

A Guide to Caring for a Loved-One with Alzheimer's Disease

By Bonnie Edwards

Chapter 1

Pre-Caregiver and Post-Corporate

Okay so I am a 48 year old female working in corporate America for 30 years selling print and digital advertising first in Las Vegas and then in New Jersey.

Deadlines, goals, and numbers, along with raising my two children plus two step children, rolled through my days from start to finish. Most of the time it felt like there wasn't anytime to breath.

Never really taking time to reflect or even enjoy the fruits of my labor I kept my head down and did what I had to to do to get through the day, raise the kids and try to be a good wife after all that.

Of course there were many instances of joy over the years but it always seemed fleeting and unsustainable.

The times that I made killer bonuses or won great trips in sales contests were amazing but with all things, at some point, I would eventually top out, and my goals would be unattainable.

Not only did that happen, but so did the recession in 2008. I survived twelve company reorganizations and downsizes. With each reorganization, the workload became more and more unrealistic and achievement of any type of goal was fleeting. With this comes a great deal of stress and self-defeating self talk.

By 2017, I was burnt out, self medicating and felt closer to a mental/emotional breakdown than ever before.

So I checked myself into a rehab/wellness center in Laguna Beach, CA for a 30 day stay to get a well deserved break and some therapy to help me cope with my crumbling tower.

The amazing therapy and counseling I received there along with more clarity than I have ever had in my life turned my 30 day stay into a 60.

So after 60 days of work on myself and a clear mind and heart, I boarded a plane back home to my husband, family and career. With all the clarity I received while away I had some amazing plans for the rest of my life.

I'm sure you have all heard the phrase "God laughs while we make plans"! Well here is proof.

The morning I was to board the plane to come home and start my new amazing life, my husband called to say that his mom's house burnt down and she was with him and they would be picking me up from the airport and most likely living with us indefinitely or at least until we made a plan.

Talk about a moment of profound self searching. I can't even lie, for a moment, I considered not getting on the plane and never coming home.

But something in me had changed so much by then and I couldn't deny the call, so I just put my hands up and said "Okay

God, I will do what you want me to do instead", and headed home.

Chapter 2

Should We Keep Our Loved One At Home When They Can No Longer Live Unassisted

A candle loses nothing by lighting another candle.
~ James Keller ~

Most adult children live in denial for a long time before acknowledging that the person who has been their support system and home base their entire life is no longer able to care for themselves. Sometimes it's just a realization, and for some, like us, the unthinkable happened.

My mother-in-law's house burnt down one spring morning in 2017 (while she was at the doctor's office with my husband) due to a holy candle that was left burning under an icon. It was glaringly clear, at this point, she could no longer live alone. Sometimes when we put off things we need to take care of, God gives us a little nudge, then a shove in the right direction :)

So one moment my husband and I are empty-nesters with good jobs and plans to travel, and the next moment we are faced with the sole responsibility of caring for his mom with Alzheimer's.

Finding or providing care for a loved one with Alzheimer is one of the most difficult task you may ever encounter. If you are fortunate, your loved one has created a living will and a little direction on how they would like to live as they age. Usually this is not the case, and of course, by the time your loved one is diagnosed they are may already be unable to make major life decisions.

After weighing all the pros and cons of each potential solution and a lot of soul searching, my husband and I decided that I would leave my career of 30 years to be a full time caregiver to mom at home. At the time, it seemed like the only solution for us.

How hard could it be, I thought? She was very sweet, full of gratitude, called me her sweet beautiful lady and told many many times a day how much she loved me.   At this point in time she was also still very able to pretend to understand or remember things so it was kind of fun to have someone to hang out with that was game to do whatever you suggested. And I would get to stay home instead of going to work! What could be wrong with that!

Chapter 3

The Journey Begins

Never believe that a few caring people can't change the world.
For, indeed, thats all who ever have.
~ Margaret Mead ~

However......

the job of care taking of mom was much much harder than I

could have ever imagined.

Trust me, even if you are an extremely nurturing soul (which I'm

not) this task will take you to your limits. It is truly like caring for a

3 year old who doesn't retain any information from minute to

minute but still keeps asking the question.   Remind yourself often

that your loved one is confused, scared and disoriented. This will

keep you in the right mind set because you will have moments

where you will think you can't do this.   The poem on the next page is one I referred to often throughout our journey. This helped me to regain composure, reset my mind and carry on.

One thing I can promise you, this will be the most challenging and, by far, the most rewarding task you will ever do in your life, whether you are the caregiver type or not.

You will amaze yourself with your innate ability to provide care for someone you love, while most of the time, caring for other loved ones at the same time.

Do Not Ask Me to Remember

Do not ask me to remember,

Don't try to make me understand,

Let me rest and know you're with me.

Kiss my cheek and hold my hand.

I'm confused beyond your concept,

I am sad and sick and lost.

All I know is that I need you

To be with me at all cost.

Do not lose your patience with me,

Do not scold or curse or cry

I can't help the way I'm acting.

Can't be different though I try.

Just remember that I need you,

That the best of me is gone.

Please don't fail to stand beside me,

Love me 'til my life is done.

~ Owen Darnell ~

Lo and behold, we developed a routine that worked for both of us and settled in to our new life. Though I was sure the caption under my yearbook picture read "Least likely to be a Caregiver", I learned how to be a caregiver……..the hard way!

As with all things, I wish I would have known in the beginning the things I know now about being a caregiver. If you are already a professional caregiver…..these things may seem basic and part of your job, but if you have never had to care for a loved one with Alzheimer's…..this book is for you!

The following chapters are a story of our Alzheimer's journey with tips and tricks to make your journey easier from beginning to end. Each loved one will progress with Alzheimer's Disease in their own unique way, however I have noticed a similar vein of progression in many patients (tissue stuffing, spitting, sundowners, etc) through my own experience and activity on social media support groups for caregivers of Alzheimer patients.

Chapter 4

Shitastrophys Happen

In the beginning, most days consists of many small meals throughout the day and poop. During this stage it seemed that all I did was cook one thing after another and monitor bathroom activity.   It was like she had a bottomless stomach that she was constantly trying to fill.   No one knows for sure why this happens but it is definitely a common trait in Alzheimer's patients.   **Tip: Try cooking their favorite foods in bulk when possible and keep snacks around, but try not to fall in the habit of eating the snacks yourself :)**

Another common trait with Alzheimer's patients? ..... Various antics to hide POOP!   At this point, mom was often surprised by bowel movements and forgot that this happens.....so if no one was paying attention she would try to hide it in the corner of the bathroom, rub it on walls and floors, etc.

She also had a bad habit of "going in" when the poop did not want to come out on it's own ….. creating shitty hands.

One particular evening my husband convinced me to slip out to the sunroom for a jacuzzi bath because mom was sleeping. I knew it was a "poop" day but she looked like she was sleeping so peacefully I reluctantly agreed. And of course, when I came back in, mom had gotten up, pooped all over the bathroom floor and was rubbing it on the wall creating shitty hands! ALWAYS TRUST YOUR INSTINCTS!

And sometimes there's a bout of constipation and it just won't come out. What to do? What to do? Well if you are a rookie, like me, you will try to use a long stick to help the turd hanging out gain downward momentum. **Tip: This did work, however, through trial and error I learned if you gently massage the area just above the rectum it will help aid the movement and make your loved one feel much much better.** Odds are, until it comes out, your loved one is going to keep trying to get it out themselves.....creating shitty hands.

GET DISPOSABLE GLOVES Nothing will seem near as bad if you have gloves on. Get gloves, have baggies and paper towels stashed in suspect places.....you will need them. Once a "shitas-trophy" has happened is not the time to start looking for supplies! Also, move to pull ups as soon as your loved one will allow.

A good sense of humor can help you a great deal. Sometimes it is so hard not to take things personally and you have to remind yourself constantly ......it's not personal.   Modern medicine and science are unable to define the reasons why this disease changes our loved ones so much.......but it does!

CHAPTER 5

ALZHEIMER'S DISEASE
WHO'S EFFECTED AND TREATMENT OPTIONS

According to the Alzheimer Association, one in ten people over the age of 65 will be diagnosed with Alzheimer's Disease in 2019. This is a staggering figure considering most family structures today consist of both parents working to provide an income for their family. So when an afflicted loved one is unable to live alone, who is going to care for them? Most people affected by the disease are at least 2-5 years in before actually receiving a diagnosis. This means, most likely, that no one has planned for this type of end of life care.

Even though Alzheimer's Disease is one of the top ten causes of death, it is the only one without cure. Also, many Alzheimer's deaths are recorded as something else. In the later stages of Alzheimer's, other health conditions could develop like infections, pressure sores and hip fractures. Pneumonia and Urinary Tract Infections claim responsibility for the death of many Alzheimer's and Dementia patients.

If you are lucky, and you treat your loved one as if in a bubble, you may be able to avoid some of the things listed above.

At the moment, there are two drugs that are approved by the FDA (Food and Drug Administration):

Cholinesterase Inhibitors. According to the Mayo Clinic https://www.mayoclinic.org/diseases-conditions/alzheimers-disease/in-depth/alzheimers/art-20048103) one way Alzheimer's disease harms the brain is by decreasing levels of a chemical messenger (acetylcholine) that's important for alertness, memory, thought and judgment. Cholinesterase (ko-lin-ES-tur-ays) inhibitors boost the amount of acetylcholine available to nerve cells by preventing its breakdown in the brain. Below are three cholinesterase inhibitors that are commonly prescribed:

- **Donepezil (Aricept)** is approved to treat all stages of the disease. It's taken once a day as a pill.

- **Galantamine (Razadyne)** is approved to treat mild to moderate Alzheimer's. It's taken as a pill once a day or as an extended release capsule twice a day.

- **Rivastigmine (Exelon)** is approved for mild to moderate Alzheimer's disease. It's taken as a pill. A skin patch is available that can also be used to treat severe Alzheimer's disease.

Memantine (Namenda) is approved by the FDA for treatment of moderate to severe Alzheimer's disease. The Mayo Clinic states that it works by regulating the activity of glutamate, a messenger chemical widely involved in brain functions — including learning and memory. It's taken as a pill or syrup. Common side effects include dizziness, headache, confusion and agitation.

A combination of **Donepezil** and **Memantine (Namzaric)** is also available and approved by the FDA in a capsule form.

The reason I'm sharing all this medical stuff is because it will be ultimately up to you to find the right mix of medication based on how each medication affects your loved one. At some point you will also have to decide when the medication is no longer making a difference and stop administering.

The right decision regarding the care of a loved one will be vastly different for each family. The biggest and most glaring issue with Alzheimer's Disease is your loved one can have the best health insurance money can buy but if their diagnosis is Alzheimer's Disease their insurance will provide little to no help paying for their care. Alzheimer's care is considered babysitting in the healthcare industry and not of medical nature ….. and it's just not entirely true.

Of course they will pay for visits to the neurologist, general practitioner, podiatrist, Alzheimer's medication, etc. However, no money is allocated for home health aids or visiting nurses/doctors which you so desperately need. If you want that, you have to pay out of pocket. Or, you can persuade one of your loved one's health care providers to deem them home-bound and unable to leave the house. This is tricky, however, because if the doctor does this, he definitely loses a patient. Be persistent with all medical care professionals involved to get the right care, if you just follow along, like we did in the beginning, you will end up frustrated and worn out.

And don't forget, all those professionals listed above are more than happy to send you and your loved one running around for blood work, ultrasounds, scans …. you name it … if your insurance will pay for it …they will order it!   This will leave you holding a bag of shit in a doctor's office, *literally*!

If your loved one had the insight to purchase long term healthcare then you have a hope and a prayer of assistance on your journey. If not, you are on your own until you get to hospice care which could be years down the line.

Caring for a loved one with Alzheimer's Disease requires a lot more than a good bed side manner. Sometimes your loved one will do things so far out of character that you may find yourself wondering if they are doing it on purpose. Trust me, they are not. They are lost and trapped in a terrifying nightmare. THIS WILL TEST YOUR PATIENCE! As the caregiver you have to find a source of constant reminders that they do not know what they are doing.

Most of us never even dreamed that we would be taking care of a loved one with a terminal disease, especially one that makes no sense.. Not just for you, but everyone in your immediate family and inner circle will be affected. From children who still live at home to friends you have no time to see, annual events, holidays, etc., everything will be affected.

I only emphasize this to hopefully give you a head start on a positive mindset for this journey because at the end of the day, it is truly rewarding caring for a loved one in their time of need.

In the beginning Mom was in her own room. This did not last long as she would wake up several times at night and start searching for people. I would often wake up to her standing over me. She was terrified to be alone so for her safety and our own sanity we moved her into our bedroom.

Sounds sexy......right!

For us, the task at hand of taking care of mom and our great desire for a good nights sleep over-ruled our desire for privacy as a married couple.

This was much more comfortable for Mom and for the most part we started to get a decent night's sleep. But of course, not without some humming, singing and several declarations of love for "her beautiful lady" ..... that was me, throughout the night. And many trips to the ladies room.

Tissue stuffing was also a huge issue at this point and they would literally fly out of shirt sleeves, underwear, socks and most often they weren't clean, if you know what I mean! Even though this drove us crazy we tried to find a little humor in it by offering a tissue from mom's pant leg should someone sneeze.

Most days she was able to use the restroom on her own with a little help cleaning up and still eating food on her own. This is when you may think that you have everything under control and maybe you can breath. But then you noticed that your loved one is sucking the flavor off their food, spitting back out on the plate and re-eating it. Sounds too gross ….. But wait, there is more, she also loved Lays potato chips but began putting the sucked chips back in the bag……..yuuucck!

To this day, no one at my house will eat out of a bag of chips unless they see it being opened.

Chapter 6

All the Questions and Finding Diversions

Some people care too much.
I think it's called love.
~ Winnie The Pooh ~

Get in the mind set to answer the same questions over and over.
If your loved one gets stuck on something, try to divert their attention by mentioning anything else. This will usually jar them off the banter for awhile.

Try not to use phrases like "Do You Remember" or "Did You Forget". In the beginning stages most sufferers do not realize they have a disease and are often embarrassed that they can't remember and may withdraw from the activity.

Some will feel like people around the house are taking things from them, even you! Diversion is the only way I found to diffuse this type of situation, that and showing my loved one her shoes that she was convinced just walked out the door on my daughter's feet. Like I said, at first it's a little unsettling but once you understand more you start to find humor in each situation.

For my mother-in-law, she always wanted to go home or go to church, as she lived on church property and was able to walk to church daily for 30 years. When she became insistent I would put her in the car and take her for a drive or walk around the neighborhood (telling her the whole time we were on our way to church) until she would get tired. The more physical activity you can get your loved one to do, the better.

Items with bright colors or very shiny or sparkly seem to be attractive, along with word searches, puzzles, match games will help entertain for awhile.

On good days my husband and I would take her out to do something fun. She was able to go putt putt golfing, cruise boating on the lake, music outings, etc. Every Sunday, as he did for years, my husband would take her to church. This was her favorite thing of all.

All of this is fun and its wonderful to spend time with your loved one until a "shitastrophy" happens…..AND IT WILL!

Remember the surprise bowel movements? …….Well they will happen….in the store, at the doctor's office, in the car, in the restaurant, at church.

Tip: Be prepared!   Always travel with a bag of supplies; paper towels, new clothes/shoes, diapers and baby wipes.   You are definitely going to need them at some point.

This disease will progress no matter how hard you try to stop it. Being prepared for a "shitatrohpy" will help you enjoy time with your loved one and make you feel more confident leaving the house.

Chapter 7

Doctor's Appointments and Medication

Doctors appointments are always fun.

Here's the deal, at this point in the disease, the doctor is pretty much getting the information from you because mom continually answers all questions with a laugh and "I wasn't thinking about that".

Not to mention how basic the questions are. What is your name? How old are you? What year is it? This is the extent of your loved one's neurologist appointment once a diagnosis has been made.

So really, a huge waste of time and energy! Alzheimer's meds do slow the progression of this disease but it is still merely a guessing game what works for each patient.   Even though science is working daily to find meds that are truly effective at slowing or even curing the disease, today there isn't one. Wouldn't it be a miracle if there was "a little pill" that worked for everyone suffering from Alzheimer's, but the glaring fact is …… THERE ISN'T!

Pay close attention to your loved one to make sure they are not getting to much of something. You will know it's too much if they become lethargic, lose their balance, refuse to get up or move. It will be highly up to you to monitor this. Each visit to the Neurologist consists of a few questions from the doctor and a new prescription.

As the one who spends the most time with your loved one, you will basically have to monitor and adjust as needed, of course, within the guidelines of the doctor.   If you tell the doctor that your loved one is more agitated, more sleepy, more confused, less interested…..basically any of those things…..they will adjust the meds and usually up because there is no other option. No further tests are done to see if any effort is helping or slowing the progression, so it really is up to you.

Don't be afraid of anti-psychotic/anti-anxiety meds like Seraquil and Lorazepam. At some point your loved one may experience sun-downers, which is a condition where they become extremely unsettled and upset as evening approaches. It's way better to find a way to calm them down than to let them get agitated and hurt themselves or even you. It's all about keeping your loved one safe, settled and comfortable.

Until there is a cure or a solid treatment plan, comfort care is all we have :(

Chapter 8

Old Habits Die and New Ones Begin

So mom stopped stuffing tissues everywhere. That's amazing, right! What new habit did she put in to play? You know what they say, "when one door closes, another one opens! Well behind the next door was spitting. Spitting Everywhere! On the floor, the couch, the bed, the vegetables at the grocery store, on the church floor, everywhere.

This was a whole new phase and a battle I never was able to win : (

If this habit develops, you will definitely go to less public places! You will also begin a love affair with carpet/furniture shampooers and paper towels and bleach…..lots of bleach! Keeping in mind that your loved one "knows not what they do" will help you deal.

In this phase, paper towels, bleach and a good carpet shampooer will be your best friends.

Trust me, I tried giving her a cup to spit in…..she would spit in the cup and then try to drink it…..not trying to be gross…..it just is. I also tried giving her a handkerchief to spit into, she would just stuff it in her sleeve and spit on the floor.

The only meager advise I have in this area is try to contain your loved one to a special seat on the couch and at the table to run damage control and where slippers or shoes. Always where slippers or shoes! You don't want to find out where to clean by stepping in it. Also turn the lights on if you are walking the normal path….it will help!

Another issue to be mindful of is having any kind of cleaner or toxic liquids sitting around, especially if its a pretty color blue or something. Your loved one will try to drink it! To them it looks like Gatorade.   It's important to keep this stuff put away.

Try to avoid having tables and furniture with sharp corners. Alzheimer's patients tend to lose their balance without warning and fall.   It's worth the extra effort to lessen the chance of acci- dent. Once your loved one has a broken limb, it is extremely hard to bounce back.

At this point, your loved one may still like to drink or even smoke. This is an area where you will need to use caution.   Alcohol for an Alzheimer's patient on meds should come with a label reading…. May cause Falls, Extreme Anger or Agitation or Happiness or a "Shitastrophy". Any and all of those things can happen!

You can try to substitute their favorite drink with juice or mixers to limit consumption if this is something they still find joy in.   This is a personal thought, but at this stage of the game, I think you should allow your loved one whatever they want as long as you can keep them safe! I don't think a glass of wine or a cigarette is

going to change anything.

Chapter 9

UTI'S (Urinary Tract Infections)

URINARY TRACT INFECTIONS - UTI"s are so common in Alzheimer patients and can have a devastating effect on your loved one. Be on the look out for the signs so that you can start antibiotics right away.

Some of the more obvious things to look for are listed below:

- Change in behavior
- Inconsolable
- Obvious pain in abdomen
- Smelling urine
- Frequent urination

Lots of fluids and keeping the potty area clean can help a lot to avoid UTI's but they are going to happen. Unfortunately, this can not be diagnosed without a trip to the doctor. You will make this trip with your loved one several times before the doctor will see it as re-occuring. Get your doctor to put multiple refills of antibiotic on file so you can get them immediately upon realizing you are dealing with a UTI. If you have to wait till morning when the Doctor's office opens to get a prescription …. You are in for a long night!

If your loved one is still able to swallow pills, a stronger antibiotic can be administered. If you need it in a liquid form it will still work but it will definitely be less effective. The good news is the liquid form tastes like bubble gum so your loved one will most likely like the taste. You should notice a marked improvement in your loved one within forty eight hours of the first dose.

If you have ever experienced a UTI, IT'S VERY PAINFUL! Get antibiotics as soon as you recognize the signs. If the doctor insists on checking the urine before prescribing antibiotics, explain your loved one's condition and ask if you can drop off a urine sample to forego bringing your loved one out when they do not feel good.

Tip: Remember, as caregiver, you are their voice. If you don't speak up on these occasions, no one can.

Chapter 10

When Your Loved One No Longer
Leaves The House

There will come a time when your loved one will no longer be able to leave the house and that means you can't either. If your loved one is still cognitive enough to do a craft, put together puzzles or read ..... this will help, but even that will make you stir crazy after awhile.

It may seem like your loved one doesn't enjoy doing puzzles, coloring or crafting but it's more about spending quality time. Most people who suffer from Alzheimer still like to interact with others even if they don't make sense. One of Mom's quirks was constantly making a noise which sounded like Bo, Bo, Bo, Bo, Bo,

Bo. So instead of being annoyed with the constant Bo, Bo, Boing we all started to add Bo Bo to our conversations which always made her feel like we understood and made us laugh. The most beautiful part about this is that she would always sing her bo bo bo's which made us believe that where ever she was in her head she was happy and singing.

Looking though old pictures of familiar people and things is a good way to spend time with your loved one. Hopefully this is an activity they like, some may find this type of activity to over-whelming, so pay attention. Music is often soothing but you will have to experiment with what works as their taste in music is like-ly vastly different from yours.

If your loved one is still mobile, walking outside is an awesome activity and no one cares if they spit in the grass!

Playing yard games outside is a great way to add sunshine to both of your lives. Summer will definitely be a better time for both you and your loved one if you live in a colder region, like New Jersey.

If your loved one is capable and wants to do things around the house, by all means, get them a broom. They want something to do just as much as you do. Obviously you can't count on a job well done but your loved one will feel like they are contributing.

This is the time when family members and people close to your loved one will come in handy. You can no longer take your loved one to the the store and out to run errands but they still have to be done, Right?

How this pans out is largely going to depend on your support system. The less independent your loved one becomes, the less comfortable others are pitching in and hanging out while you go out and do some errands. If you can afford hired aids for this, great! For us, living on one income did not afford this. Sometimes you will be frustrated and mad because you feel no one wants to help but you have to remember your immediate family is dealing with this in their own way also and may be extremely un-comfortable with the responsibility.

It's funny, some will stop answering your calls because even though on the surface the conversation sounds like this…..”Do you think you could hang out with mom while I run out and do some errands”, but what they really hear is …. “While I'm out, Mom may have a “shitastrophy”and since I'm not home, you will have to clean it up yourself”. Who could really blame anyone for not answering…..LOL!

Chapter 11

General Hygiene

Underwear vs Diapers/Pull-ups

You will have to help your loved one make the transition from their regular underwear to pull ups. As the disease progresses they have a hard time knowing when they need to go and often wait until its too late to head that way. Pull ups will save you countless clean up hours and now they are so stylish your loved one may not even know the difference.

Tip: Chucks/bed pads are a necessity in the latter stages. It's much easier to remove a soiled pad than to change all the bedding.

Showering and Hygiene

This is always a difficult area to delve into. Depending again on their mobility, using the shower is easiest and eventually you will need to add shower chair for safety. There is only one thing that an Alzheimer's patient is more scared of than being alone and that is getting undressed, especially by someone other than themselves.

More than once I found myself in a full on tug of war with my mother in law and a shitty nightgown! It starts with innocent re-moval, then she claps down on it, then you think you are stronger, so you give it a yank, but she holds on now even tighter....THAT'S WHEN YOU REALIZE WHAT YOU ARE DOING!

After some trial and error, I found soft coaxing and the promise of a place in the shower where it was warm worked.... Most of the time! Once they are in a shower chair you will definitely need a removable shower head to help with cleaning up a real "shitas-trophy" and for general bathing, but definitely for "shitastrophies".

Following up a shower with a warm robe from the dryer will definitely put your loved one at ease and make it easier to get them dressed and their hair combed and dry.

As Alzheimer's Disease progresses it becomes increasingly difficult to keep your loved one clean without violating their privacy but it is so important that their private area is kept as clean as possible to avoid infections and sores.

Bed sores and pressure sores will also be a pain point for both you and your loved one.
Use pillows, special pads and air-bubble mattresses to minimize pressure. If your loved one is still mobile make sure they are moving around every 15 minutes to a half hour, if they are bedridden try changing their position every 2 hours or so.

Stage 1 sores should be treated with mild soap and water and covered with a moisture barrier to protect the skin from further damage.

Stage 2 sores should be cleaned with salt water (saline) to remove loose dead tissue. Do not use hydrogen peroxide or iodine cleanser as they can damage the skin.

Stage 3 and up sores will need to be treated by a physician. Usually an antibiotic will be prescribed to help with the infection along with a medicated moisture barrier.

Obviously, keeping your loved ones undergarments clean and dry will also be key. Even if you do all this and more, pressure and bed sores are likely to happen. Don't beat yourself up about it!

Chapter 12

When Is It Time For Hospice Services?

The general thought people have when hospice is mentioned is that it is the end of life for your loved one, but this is far from the truth. Hospice is wonderful resource to utilize in helping you care for your loved one in the best possible way. The biggest hurdle you have to jump is signing a DNR - Do Not Recessitate. Just the thought of this makes you feel like a failure or like you are giving up but to prolong suffering seems somehow inhumane.

The truth in the light of day is.....your loved one is not going to be getting better and Alzheimer's is an incurable disease. Your loved one qualifies for these services as long as they have an Alzheimer's diagnosis and is no longer seeking life saving measures like (surgery, new trial drugs, etc). Your loved one could be on hospice for years before the end of life.

And remember, it is still very much up to you if you would like to continue to administer Alzheimer's medication or antibiotics. Hospice will once again caution against it but if you feel your loved one is still benefiting from the medicine, give it to them. As mentioned earlier, they may not pay for the meds but you can definitely administer them.

Do yourself a favor and get the help! If nothing else, you will learn some great tips about caring for your loved one and even get a little time for yourself. They will provide you with a comfort pack filled with different medications to promote comfort (pain medication, suppositories, anti-depressants, and morphine). These medications are provided to keep your loved one comfortable at all times. They provide all the supplies you need to care for your loved one at home. Diapers, chucks/pee pads, gloves, body wash and lotion and any type of medication prescribed by hospice doctor like Seraquel or Lorazapham. This is a huge money-saving bonus because at this point you will be using all those things on the reg.

Hospice will also provide respite care for your loved one in a skilled nursing facility for up to five days for every ninety days your loved one is on hospice. This varies state to state so please check with your local Alzheimer chapter. This can be an amazing perk and you will need a break to rejuvenate and do self care.

A WORD TO THE WISE ......

Even though your hospice team will assure you that they have everything covered and you should just relax and take it easy, do your due diligence.

After your loved one arrives at a facility for a respite stay......GO THERE! Give them a little time to get your loved one settled in and then go there with the comfort care pack and sign it in with a supervisor and go over how your loved one needs to be cared for.

Does your loved one still get up to use the restroom? Do they wander? Can they take pills or do they need to be crushed?

Does your loved one eat food, puree'd food or nutritional shakes? It is best to bring a typed up sheet of care that your loved one will require and tape it to the wall in their room.

Nursing home staff changes often so you can never assume they know the specifics about your loved one, even if they have been there in the past. Also, it's good idea to let staff know that family members along with hospice staff will be stopping in to check up, this will keep them on their toes and give you a little piece of mind. This is your time to rest but try to get family members to drop in for a visit. I'm sure you have all heard a horror story about a nursing home before :(

On the day your loved one is coming home, go back to facility and get your loved one's suitcase and comfort care pack. I can just tell you there is a lot of suspicious behavior going on around the comfort care pack because it contains morphine so I would air on the side of caution regarding it. If it comes up missing during transport of your loved one to and from the facility......it's a blame game. The facility blames the transport drivers, the hospice nurse blames the facility or worse case scenario ….. they blame you!

Should You Give Your Loved Ones Antibiotics Once Hospice Is Involved?

Giving antibiotics to your loved one in the end stages is considered prolonging life to some. To me, it provides comfort and relief from infection, especially a UTI (Urinary Tract Infection). Just remember, the decision is ultimately yours. Hospice will caution against it and a lot of time, will not pay for the prescription but do what feels right in your heart. Your loved one's GP can prescribe it.

For me, I was able to see a notable improvement within as little as 24-48 hours, so I believe antibiotics to be part of comfort care.

Once again, since your loved one may be unable to make decisions, everything is up to you!

Chapter 13

The End

You can read about it, watch documentaries, see others go through it but nothing will prepare you for the final week. I was provided with all the materials describing how my loved one would eventually not want to get out of bed anymore, and then not want to eat or drink anything but somehow I thought it would be different for us. The truth is, it happened just the way the Alzheimer's information said it would and I would be lying if I said it wasn't devastating, because it was!

Watching someone you love and cared for die is an extremely emotional process. The feeling of being helpless is overwhelming. Allow your hospice staff to guide you at this time because you will not be making rational decisions. I was feeding mom with a syringe to try to bring life back to her and my nurse explained that if she doesn't swallow the fluid she will breath it into her lungs and aspirate. This is not a peaceful way to go :(She also explained that the amount of fluids she needed would have to be administered intravenously to make any kind of difference, which is something we already decided we would not do.

Though something very amazing and beautiful happened in the final weeks. Mom would often reach up with both arms and called loved ones who have passed (mother, husband, daughter and brother) by name and ask me why they can't come closer. One day she told me that my mom was also there :) I have no doubt in my mind her loved ones and God were there to walk her home and this was a huge comfort.

My husband and I struggled in the end of when to start giving her the morphine for comfort as most of the time she did not appear to be in any kind of pain. But how can you know for sure? Often if your loved one is in pain, even if unconscious, they will clench their fingers together, but sometimes its just hard to tell. It is true that morphine can help your loved one's respiratory function better but it has also been said to aid the organs in shutting down. So you see the struggle.

But in the end, it's the end.

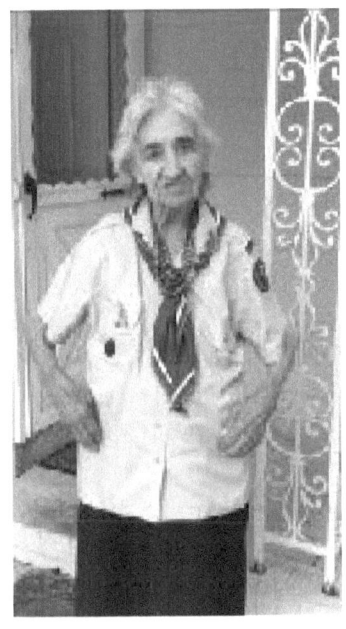

Mom passed away on Thursday, June 6, 2019. For the Russian Orthodox, this is Ascension Day, kind of like a free pass to heaven. For all of us who loved her dearly, this was such a wonderful thing and so fitting for a woman who spent her entire life as God's faithful servant. She was also a faithful and life long scout member of the Russian Scouts, created by her own husband. She was buried in her scout uniform, as requested. Once a scout, always a scout. Scouts showed up at the funeral in large numbers and fully dressed in scout attire, just like mom :)

Chapter 14

Now What?

So the funeral is over, hospice equipment removed from my bed-room and everyone goes back to their lives and busy schedules. If you are anything like me, you will expect to feel relief and a sense of freedom.   However, I felt lost and alone and I missed her so much.

I could still hear her humming in my sleep and felt her presences so strong still.   I kept expecting to walk around the corner into my bedroom and she would be there like she had been for so long. I am so happy for her that she is now at peace and at home with God, but for me the sadness and loss was unexpected and larger than life. I was struggling with what to do with my life now.

In the first weeks, I did a lot of cleaning and organizing. I was amazed at the amount of cleaning that went unnoticed by me even though I was home 24/7. Even with that I couldn't seem to get a grip on moving on, maybe getting a job or just staying locked in the house like I had been for so long, As each thought was a little overwhelming I decided to take a little trip to my best friends house in Florida for a few days for different scenery and a new perspective.

And a little self care. Read that again! And a little self care. It is so important to take care of yourself while caring for your loved one. I guess this is hindsight info, because I arrived at my friends house with over-grown hair, broken and chipped nails and tension on my face.

Hopefully you will have this person in your life to clean you up and put you back together again. Either way, please care for yourself also.

After a few days of the sun beach and self-care, I was beginning to see the light and felt more ready to face the next assignment God has in mind for me. Until then I will spend time reconnecting with family and friends and finish this book. Hopefully it will find you when you need it the most.

I know some of the things in this book do not sound like something you may want to sign up for but I promise you there were more good times than bad. Caring for a loved one is very rewarding and I have grown as a person in so many ways. I hope if you get the call, you will answer and if you do, I pray that this book will help you along the way.

www.ingramcontent.com/pod-product-compliance
Lightning Source LLC
Chambersburg PA
CBHW051400280526
45784CB00007B/3044